Understanding Contraception

A guide for
Black ladies

By Dr. Adaeze Ifezulike

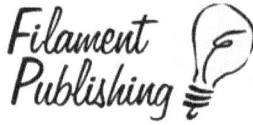

Filament
Publishing

Published by
Filament Publishing Ltd
16 Croydon Road, Waddon, Croydon,
Surrey, CRO 4PA, United Kingdom
Telephone +44 (0)20 8688 2598
Fax +44 (0)20 7183 7186
info@filamentpublishing.com
www.filamentpublishing.com

ISBN 978-1-910125-07-6

Printed by CreateSpace

Dedicated with love to my daughters,
Sonnie, Chizzy and Jewel.

The stories used in this book are based on actual patients that I have worked with in my practice as a GP. All names have been changed to preserve confidentiality.

Special thanks to Maya Angelou for permitting the use of her lovely poem, *Remembrance*.

Illustrations by Medical Illustration Unit of the University of Aberdeen.

Cartoon illustrations by Rick Coleman.

Additional illustrations by Clare Clarke at Evoke Graphic Design.

Contents

Foreword

The right to choose contraception or to become pregnant is indeed a decision often shaped by multiple factors including lack of information, religion, social and cultural norms. This makes millions of African women and girls globally unable to control their sexual lives. Choices about contraception are tangled with taboos. There is still too much silence around sexual matters and contraception in our communities.

Understanding Contraception: A guide for Black ladies fills a major gap in knowledge and should be made widely available to women from all walks of life both in the UK and all over the world.

During a training programme on sexuality with women from a London borough, I asked whether they had ever bought condoms before. The only brave woman to respond in the affirmative said this was only possible because she hid the condoms under other items when she got to the counter because she felt so shy. Such courageous women are rare within our African communities.

I am still amazed that in this internet age the myths and misconceptions cited in this booklet continue to inform and shape women's contraceptive decision-making. Dr Adaeze Ifezulike has responded to the challenges and dilemmas that she sees daily in her surgery and provides a very practical and easy to read book.

Understanding Contraception should be made widely available to Black women of all ages. I call on the NHS and women's organisations to help women gain knowledge and confidence about contraception so that they can make key decisions in their personal lives.

Knowledge is power but, over the past years, I have come to recognise that changing attitudes, taboos and social norms also requires enabling women to have confidence, to speak out and take control of their lives. It is time that Black women to be more proactive. But they need support along the way.

Contraceptive advice and the ability to safely use contraception with their partners should be a reality for all women and I wholeheartedly welcome the opportunity to be part of this new movement to enable Black women to have the right to choose contraception that meets their needs and fits in with their lives.

Naana Otoo-Oyortey MBE
Executive Director, FORWARD
FORWARD (Foundation for Women's Health Research and Development) is an African Diaspora women led UK-registered campaign and support charity dedicated to advancing and safeguarding the sexual and reproductive health and rights of African girls and women.

Introduction

One only has to think of athletes Kelly Homes and Jessica Ennis; politicians Baroness Amos, Diane Abbott and Oona King; newsreader Moira Stuart; and actresses Sophie Okonedo and Thandie Newton, to recognise the positive contributions Black British women have made to the United Kingdom.

Yet, despite these inspiring role models, Black women in Britain continue to live with the consequences of poor sexual health.

- In England and Wales in 2012, 10% of women having abortions were Black or Black British. Of these women, 49% had experienced one or more previous abortions, the highest of all ethnic groups in the UK.[1]

- A National Survey of Sexual Attitudes & Lifestyles (NATSAL) 2000 reported significantly lower contraceptive use by non-married Black African and Caribbean women compared with white women and less use of hormonal and permanent methods compared with barrier types.[2]

- Research by Marie Stopes International found women of Black or Black British ethnic origin were less likely to use a regular method of contraception.[3]

- NATSAL 2000 also reported that the number of sexual partners in a lifetime was highest among Black Caribbean

[1] https://www.gov.uk/government/uploads/system/uploads/attachment_data/file/211790/2012_Abortion_Statistics.pdf
[2] Sexana S et al, Contraception 2006; 74(3):224-33
[3] www.mariestopes.org.uk/documents

and African men. A significant association between ethnic origin and reported sexually transmitted infections in the past five years was found, with an increased risk in sexually active black Caribbean and African men.[4]

What can be done to reverse this situation? You're making a good start by reading this book.

Why should you read this book?

If one was writing the essential and desirable characteristics for a job as "Sexual well-being promoter for British Black women", Dr Ifezulike's experience would provide the model description.

She is a migrant herself, hailing from Nigeria, and a mother of three girls. She trained in general practice before developing a special interest in Sexual and Reproductive Health.

She works in both sectors in a multicultural, urban centre. She is passionate about championing sexual well being for Black British ladies and for reducing health inequalities. She draws from 15 years' experience at the front line, both as a doctor and educator.

This book will teach you about fertility control and infection prevention by wrapping sexual and reproductive facts with real-life stories from Dr Adaeze's caseload. Maybe some of the cases will remind you of friends or relatives. Maybe they'll remind you of yourself.

---

[4] Fenton KA et al, Lancet 2005; 365(9466):1246-55

Read the book, talk to your partner, friends and family, but also a trusted health professional. They are waiting with open arms to see you.

Dr Susie Logan MB ChB MD (comm.) MRCOG MFSRH
Consultant Gynaecologist
National University Hospital
Singapore
Formerly Consultant in Sexual & Reproductive Medicine
NHS Grampian
Aberdeen, Scotland, UK

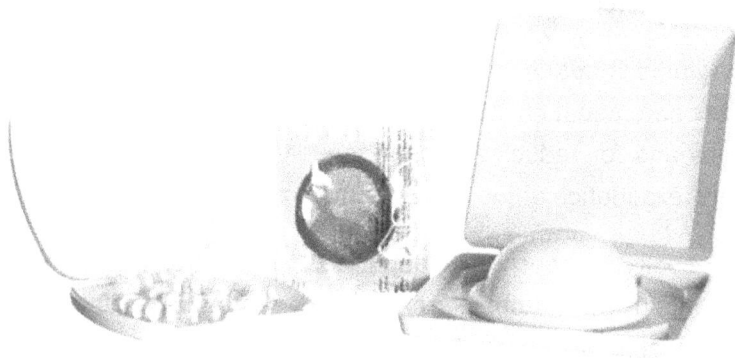

Remembrance

Your hands easy
weight, teasing the bees
hived in my hair, your smile at the
slope of my cheek. On the
occasion, you press
above me, glowing, spouting
readiness, mystery rapes
my reason.

When you have withdrawn
your self and the magic, when
only the smell of your
love lingers between
my breasts, then, only
then, can I greedily consume
your presence.

Maya Angelou

Chapter 1: The case for contraception

Amina's story

Amina looked at me, her eyes filled with tears.

"I need your help, doctor, I'm pregnant again." She paused as though the fact still amazed her, as if she was hearing the news for the first time.

I waited patiently as she fought with her emotions. When she started to speak again, the words tumbled out of her in a rush.

"It's my fifth pregnancy, doctor... we had planned to stop... we really can't afford another baby... I don't have a job and my husband's company is making people redundant so we are not sure of his job either..."

She grabbed the tissue I held out to her and dashed it to her eyes.

"I feel terrible. I had an abortion just four months ago.

"It's... we... I just can't have another baby." The tears overflowed again.

When the storm had calmed, I gently enquired what contraception she was using.

"We use condoms... Sometimes."

"At other times?"

Silence.

And then: "Nothing," she confessed.

"I just didn't think it would happen again so soon, doctor."

Fertility Fact no.1

In 2012, 49% of Black women having an abortion had a previous history of abortion. [1]

Hassana's story

Hassana had come to Aberdeen to do a Masters degree. This had been her dream for many years and when she was accepted into the programme, it looked like life couldn't get any better.

She had always been very studious with no time for boys who, she felt, were an unnecessary distraction. She was hopeful that she might get a job with one of the top oil companies in Aberdeen after acquiring her Master's degree. She spoke of her parents' pride and joy as they saw her off at the airport in Africa.

"They will be so disappointed to hear that I am pregnant," she cried in dismay.

She had become friends with a fellow student at the University and the friendship had blossomed. About four weeks prior to her coming to see me, they had sex for the very first time.

"I swear, doctor, it was only once. Just once! And I am never ever going to have sex again!" She was furious.

"I understand you feel this way now, but that may change. Perhaps we could discuss what available contraception might suit you." I started gently.

She looked at me as though she thought I was crazy and shook her head.

"Doctor, you don't understand what I am saying. I mean that I am never ever going to have sex again once I get rid of this pregnancy so I don't need contraception!"

Hassana came to see me six months later to request another termination.

Fertility Fact no. 2

If 100 sexually active women don't use contraception, 80-90% of them will become pregnant within a year.

Who is this book for?

This is for the Black African, Afro-Caribbean and Black British lady who is having sexual intercourse, does not want to get pregnant and would like information on how to avoid a pregnancy. Others, such as teenagers, mothers, counsellors, youth workers and social workers, may also find the information in this book useful.

This book recognises the prevailing cultural and religious context of the Black African and Afro-Caribbean communities which emphasises sexual abstinence for singles and frowns upon sexual activity outside of marriage.

The book respects the cultural norms of the Black community but goes further to provide critical practical information on contraception that every Black lady needs, whether single or married, sexually active or inactive.

I recognise that there may be a few women who have found themselves pregnant following rape/abuse or whose contraception has failed. This book does not cover these scenarios. However, useful contacts can be found at the end for women who find themselves in these situations.

Why is this book necessary?

There is a lack of information on contraception that specifically targets the Black woman.

This is despite the recent Department of Health Abortion statistics from England and Wales which showed a 49% rate of recurrent abortion in Black Afro-Caribbean and Black British ladies. This compares to a national rate of 36%.

In 2012, there were 203,419 abortions carried out in Great Britain. At an estimated cost of £680 per abortion[2], the cost to the National Health Service (NHS) is staggering.

But my worries are for the women themselves: what about the indirect costs to them? What about the stress of experiencing an abortion, or even multiple abortions?

And apart from the emotional trauma, what about practical problems such as needing to take time away from study or work to attend clinics, undergo the procedure and to recover afterwards? What about the mothers who need to make – and pay for – childcare arrangements?

If there is a problem in subsequent pregnancies, women often blame themselves. I have known women who see any later adverse life event as a punishment for the termination.

What is the solution?

I advocate the use of effective contraception to prevent unwanted pregnancies. I believe that all the sadness, difficulty and hardship that come with abortion can be avoided if effective contraception is used. If this book helps you to carefully consider the subject of contraception then I will be happy.

If you then go a step further and use an effective method of contraception, then my job is done.

Why listen to me?

I am a mum of three and an African living in the UK. I am a UK-trained family physician/General Practitioner and a Member of the Royal College of General Practitioners (MRCGP).

I acquired the Diploma in Sexual and Reproductive Health (DFSRH) from the Royal College of Obstetricians and Gynaecologists because I am passionate about promoting sexual health among my fellow Black women. I have letters of competence in providing all of the contraceptive methods available in the UK.

Having worked at the Centre for Sexual and Reproductive Healthcare in Aberdeen and as a GP in an urban region, I have helped ladies just like you for many years.

It is painful to see the despair of those ladies who are about to terminate an unplanned pregnancy. From my experience, abortion is never an easy decision and, all too frequently, comes with the added burdens of guilt and regret.

This book is my attempt to help Black women struggling with the issues of unplanned pregnancies, abortions and contraception.

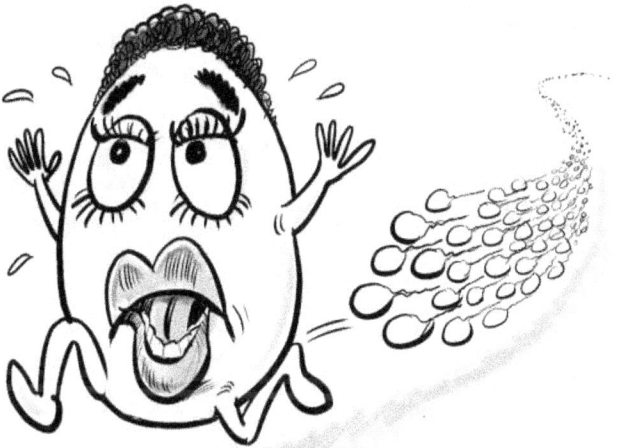

'Run! The sperms are coming!'

Chapter 2: Ill-conceived – misconceptions about contraception

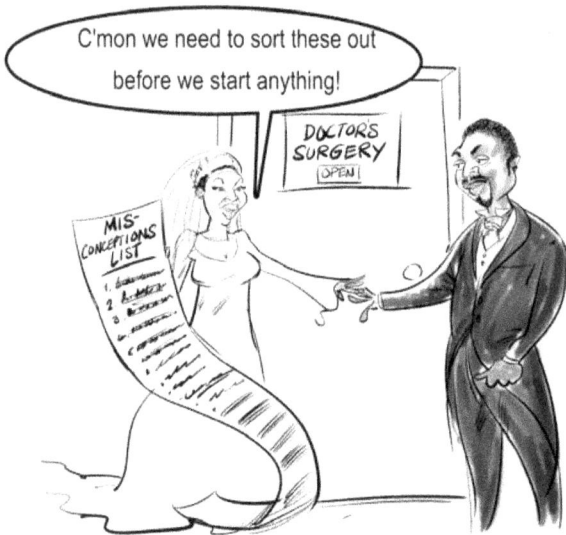

Teru's story

I went to visit Teru five weeks after the birth of her fourth child. I had got to know her through a friend and had been invited to join the family in celebrating their newest addition.

The party was in full swing at my arrival. I saw lots of old pals and it was a while before I finally located Teru in the room where she was breastfeeding the little one.

"Congratulations," I said as I handed over the gift rattles I had bought for the baby.

"Thanks," Teru smiled as she cleaned off specks of milk from the child's lips and passed her to me.

"What a gorgeous baby," I exclaimed. She was indeed a pretty thing and though her eyes were closed, she smiled broadly as though she understood she was being admired.

Teru lay back in bed; she looked exhausted but content.

"I guess we will be back in nine months to celebrate number five," I teased.

"Nooooo! This is the last one. We really must stop now!"

"So you are on contraception?"

"Not really."

"So no more sex then..."

"You know that's not possible!" She giggled.

"Ok then – what are you going to do to stop number five from coming?"

"What can one do?" she replied with a hint of helplessness.

"What about contraception?" I asked again.

"But sister, those things are bad..."

"Bad?"

"Are they not poisons?"

It took a lot of discussion to explore her concerns and fear of contraception.

Teru is not alone. It is surprising and worrying to discover just how many Black people believe that contraception is evil and has been designed by the 'white man' to limit procreation. Many Black ladies come from large families themselves. In the past, due to disease and poor health and living conditions, it was seen to be prudent to have many children with the hope that some at least would survive.

As health conditions improved, fewer children died. Yet even though this concern faded, there was no corresponding change in behaviour. It was as though people didn't understand that they could now plan their families: deciding on how many children they wanted and knowing that those children would survive.

Suddenly, we realised we didn't have to have so many babies but fell into the vacuum of not knowing how to stop having children.

As with anything 'foreign', contraception is still viewed with suspicion even among the highly educated.

Sosina's story.

Sosina had a dark secret. She had done something in the past that she felt she must be punished for forever. There was no way out for her. The guilt of her action plagued her by day and tormented her by night. She was the outcast, the sinner, the unclean!

Feelings of worthlessness were her constant companions. If I complimented her looks, she felt I was mocking her. If I asked her opinion about anything, she reacted with suspicion. If she failed a job interview, she put it down to her karma. She was never to succeed, destined always to fail.

It took many months of friendship to tease it out of her, this terrible secret. I almost laughed, nay, fainted with relief when she finally came out with it.

She had had an abortion. The big 'A'.

I didn't want to make light of her beliefs. My concern was how to ensure that what she and many others regard as The SIN didn't have to happen again. We talked about contraception. She had been brought up to regard abortion as sin but never taught how to avoid getting pregnant in the first place.

When I talk to Black women who believe that abortion is a sin and contraception is evil, we invariably come to the conclusion that no matter your belief and how you see it, contraception is always the better option.

Below are some of other concerns that women have raised with me about contraception.

Contraception makes you fat.

Only the contraceptive injection has research-based evidence of weight gain. Weight gain can be controlled by eating smaller food portions, fruits and vegetables and exercising regularly.

Contraception stops your period from coming out and the blood accumulates inside.

Hormonal contraception actually thins the lining of the womb. This means that you have little or no lining to shed during your period. There is no blood accumulating inside you.

Contraception can make you infertile.

Not true! All the contraceptives discussed in this book, apart from sterilisation, are reversible and your fertility returns when you come off them. The contraceptive injection is the only method that can delay the return of your fertility. Contraceptives that prevent ovulation (an egg being released) actually protect against conditions that reduce fertility such as ovarian cysts, fibroids and endometriosis.

Contraceptive coils can *only* be fitted in women who have delivered babies vaginally.

Both types of intrauterine devices can be fitted in women of all ages, whether they have had a vaginal delivery or not.

Contraceptive coils cause ectopic pregnancy.

You are more likely to have an ectopic pregnancy if you do not use contraception.

Douching can stop you getting pregnant.

Douching is the practice of washing out the vagina. It has **no** contraceptive benefit and can actually cause harm as the washing changes the normal environment of the vagina which is usually slightly acidic. When this acid environment is disturbed, bugs begin to grow and this leads to infection. The vagina has the ability to clean itself and simple rinsing with water is usually sufficient to keep it clean.

I cannot get pregnant if I have sex during my period.

Yes you can! Sperm can survive inside a woman for up to seven days after sex and that can be enough time for you to ovulate.

If my partner pulls out of my vagina before he ejaculates, I will not get pregnant.

Some sperm comes out of the penis even before ejaculation. Also even if he ejaculates just outside your vagina, sperm can swim inside your vagina and go on to fertilise an egg. It only takes one sperm!

If we have sex standing up or with me on top, I won't get pregnant.

Whatever position you have sex in, if sperm is released, you can still get pregnant. Sperm are great swimmers... even against gravity!

I won't get pregnant if this is my first time of having sex.

Pregnancy can result even if it is your first time.

I won't get pregnant since I am breastfeeding.

This can work if you meet the following three conditions:

1. You are exclusively breastfeeding.

2. Your periods haven't started again.

3. You are within six months of having your baby.

Helpful Hint
If you absolutely do not want to get pregnant, it's best to use contraception while you are breastfeeding.

Chapter 3: The female reproductive tract demystified!

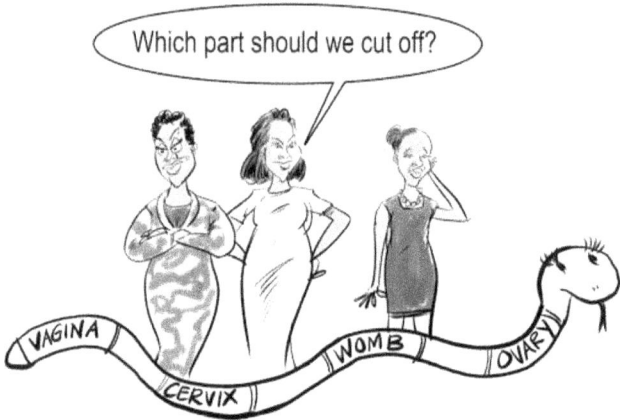

Fertility Fact no. 3

A woman has approximately one million eggs in her ovaries at birth.

Have you heard or read about the vagina (birth canal), cervix (neck of the womb), uterus (womb), and fallopian tubes (oviduct/ egg tube)?

Well, these are just names given to the different parts of a long pipe which starts with an egg (or, rarely, eggs) being released from the ovary and finishing with either menstrual blood or a baby leaving the body. Each part of the long tube (or reproductive tract) is specifically designed for its function.

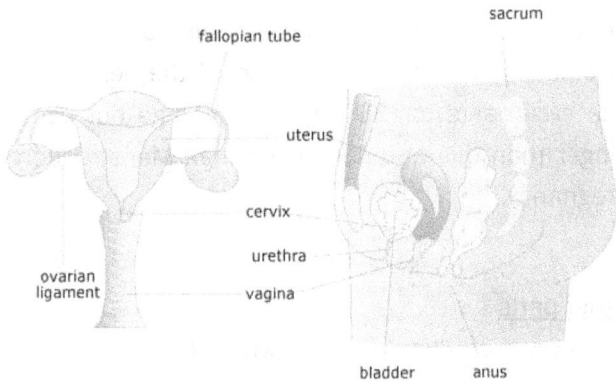

Usually one egg is released from one ovary each month and is picked up by the fallopian tube for transport to the womb. The sperm, meanwhile, swims up through the cervix and into the uterus after sex. If an egg meets a sperm in the fallopian tube, an embryo (foetus, baby) results. This process is called fertilisation.

While an egg can only survive for 24 hours once it has been released from the ovary, sperm can survive for up to seven days inside a woman.

Menstruation

Oestrogen and progesterone are female hormones which help to set up the womb to receive a fertilised egg. Their levels are high during the time the egg is moving towards the womb, thickening its lining. If the egg is not fertilised, the levels of both hormones fall and this lining breaks down and is flushed out of the body (menstruation or period).

Menstrual cycle

The first day of menstruation (when blood is first seen) is called day one. It is also referred to as the date of the Last Menstrual Period (LMP). A woman's menstrual cycle dates from this first day of bleeding up until the first day of the next round of bleeding. The cycle lasts for 28 days on average but can be shorter or longer than this and still be normal. Menstruation stops during pregnancy.

Other parts

The cervix produces mucus which helps the sperm get to the waiting egg. Later, it keeps a pregnancy in place, thinning and opening at the time of labour to allow delivery of the baby.

The vagina is the muscular outer end of the reproductive tract where the penis deposits sperm during sexual intercourse. It expands greatly during labour to allow the baby to be born.

All the organs mentioned above respond to the female hormones oestrogen and progesterone. It is the effect of these hormones on the reproductive tract that make them useful as contraceptives.

How the different contraceptions work

Barrier methods: Condoms, caps and diaphragms

As the name suggests, these act as a barrier to prevent sperm from meeting up with the egg.

Copper coil/IUD

1. Copper is toxic to both sperm and eggs and so prevents fertilisation.

2. The presence of the copper changes the secretions at the cervix and this makes it difficult for sperm to enter the cervix.

3. The copper also affects the womb lining and makes it unlikely to accept a pregnancy.

Intrauterine System (IUS, Mirena® coil)

1. Thins the lining of the womb thereby making it unlikely to accept a pregnancy.

2. Thickens the cervical mucus and makes it difficult for sperm to get into the womb.

3. In some cycles, the hormone coil stops ovulation (egg release is prevented).

Pills, patches and rings

1. Stop you producing eggs.

2. Thins the lining of the womb.

3. Thicken the secretion at the neck of the womb so that sperm cannot get in.

Progesterone only pill/mini-pill

- Thickens cervical secretions, so that they form a plug which stops sperm from getting into the womb.

- Some also inhibit ovulation so no eggs are produced.

Contraceptive injection

1. Stops you producing an egg (inhibits ovulation).

2. Thins the lining of the womb.

3. Thickens the secretions at the neck of the womb so that sperm cannot reach the egg.

Contraceptive implant

1. Inhibits ovulation (stops you producing an egg).

2. Thins the lining of the womb.

3. Thickens the secretions at the neck of the womb so that sperm cannot get in.

Female Sterilisation

The tubes that carry the eggs are tied, clipped or blocked in order to prevent the transfer of eggs down the tube or sperm from travelling up the tube.

Male sterilisation (vasectomy)

The tubes that carry sperm are cut under local or general anaesthesia so that when a man ejaculates, the fluid no longer contains sperm and so cannot fertilise a woman's eggs.

Fertility Fact no. 4

There are about 500 million sperms in 5mls of a man's ejaculate. Only one sperm is needed to fertilise an egg.

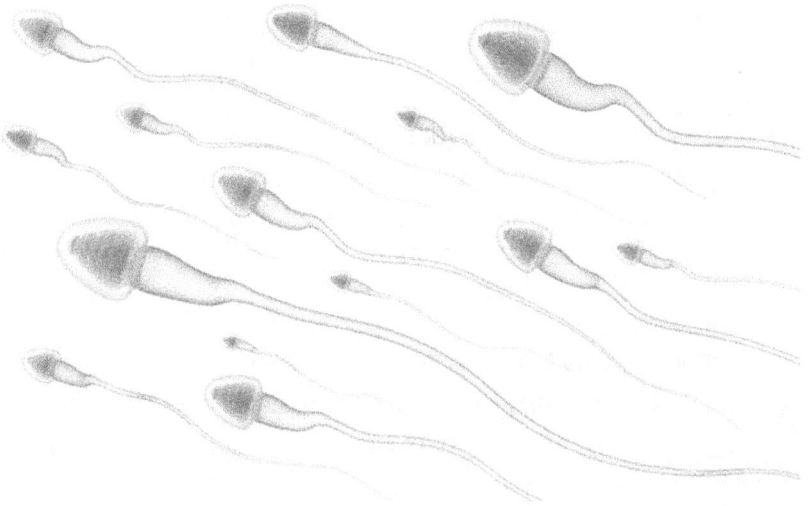

Chapter 4: Reasons for contraception

Ola's story

Ola and her husband came to see me to request contraception. She'd delivered her son six weeks before and they both felt they needed at least three years' break before any further pregnancies.

After discussing the different methods, they settled for the progesterone-only contraceptive implant which gives cover for three years and is immediately reversible. Ola could also start using it straightaway as it is safe to use during breastfeeding.

SPACING one's family might be a reason to practice effective contraception.

> **Fertility Fact no. 5**
> More than half of women who take birth control pills take them for other health benefits.[3]

Thembe's story

Thembe had had a very difficult pregnancy. She has a heart condition which makes it medically challenging to cope with pregnancy and, after the birth, her obstetrician advised that she shouldn't have any more babies.

She and her husband, however, were reluctant to do anything permanent like sterilisation. After considering several contraceptive options, they requested an intrauterine device (IUD, coil) which gives contraceptive cover for 10 years.

PRESERVING YOUR HEALTH can be an excellent reason for contraception. In some cases it is best to use contraception until one is healthier or to permanently prevent pregnancy if the risks are too great.

Jane's story

Jane, a 16-year-old, attended the clinic with her mother complaining of very heavy and painful periods, which she had suffered from since the age of 13. She used up to eight sanitary towels a day and had needed a blood transfusion at one point as she had become so anaemic and weak after a period.

After going through her medical history, I suggested a trial of contraceptive pills even though she wasn't sexually active. Other options included the injection or the hormonal coil.

The combined contraceptive pills dramatically reduced her blood flow during periods and also made them less painful. She also saved money on buying sanitary towels.

So contraceptive hormonal medication can be used for **MEDICAL REASONS** even in women who are not sexually active.

Nthabiseng's story

Twenty-eight year old Nthabiseng had just got married. She and her partner planned to go abroad for a year to undertake some further studies and wanted to use contraception as they did not want children until they had got their degrees.

She had no health problems, felt she would not be able to remember to take tablets daily and declined the injection and 'anything' going in her womb. I offered a contraceptive implant which could be removed any time with immediate return of fertility.

DELAYING PREGNANCY might be a reason to use contraception.

Adaobi's story

Adaobi, a 24-year-old lady, wept as she told me that she was in a relationship with a man who regularly abused her physically. She was making plans to leave the relationship, but was terrified she might fall pregnant before she left him.

Her partner had previously thrown out her birth control pills and she was afraid that he would notice an implant or even pull out a coil! She was relieved to learn about the contraceptive injection which she could get every three months without leaving any obvious physical signs.

SAFETY ISSUES may make it necessary to avoid pregnancy.

These are just some examples from my clinic. Other medical uses for contraception include:

- To stabilise irregular periods.

- To reduce mid-cycle/ovulation and menstrual pain.

- To ease or stop premenstrual symptoms. (Some ladies experience severe mood changes, abdominal pains or bloating and breast tenderness before their periods).

- To treat endometriosis. This distressing condition causes pain/cramps during periods and pain during sex. It is due to the presence of tissues that are normally found only inside the womb being present in other parts of the body, such as the ovaries or pelvic cavity.

- To reduce the bleeding and other effects of fibroids (benign lumps found in the womb).

- To protect against non-cancerous ovarian cysts and breast disease.

- Protection from cancers of the colon, womb and ovary.

- To improve skin problems, such as spots and pimples.

- To stop or diminish severe headaches during periods.

Fertility Fact no. 6

Contraceptive use among married women aged 15-49 in West Africa is only 14% compared to 80% in Northern Europe.[4]

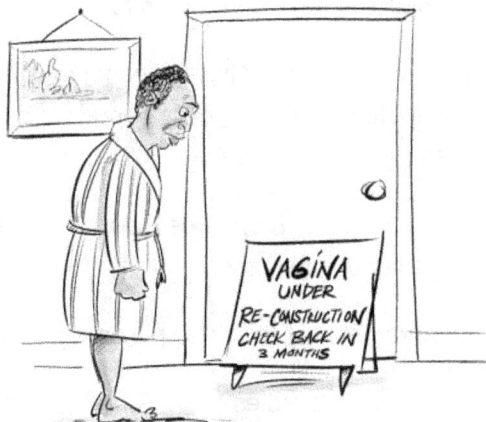

Chapter 5: Coils, pills, implants, injections, caps or what??!!

> **Fertility Quote**
> British playwright and essayist George Bernard Shaw called the rubber condom the *"greatest invention of the nineteenth century."*

It can be very confusing when it comes to contraceptive choice. But life is all about choices. Try deciding on a dress for the end of year office party – it can take the whole year!

Don't be put off by the variety of contraceptives out there. It's actually a good thing because it means that if one doesn't suit you there are plenty of other options.

The following questions can help you make your choice:

- Have you ever had children?

- Would you like to have children in future?

- Do you have any of the following conditions at the moment: Heavy bleeding during your period? Painful periods? Premenstrual symptoms? Acne?

- Would your family or friends be upset if they knew that you were using contraception?

- Would you remember to take a pill daily?

- Are you scared of needles?

- Would an injection suit you best?

- Or an implant under the skin in your arm?

- How difficult would it be for you to have genital contact in order to use a contraceptive method?

Further information can be found at http://www.fpa.org.uk/contraception-help/my-contraception-tool/ and http://www.brook.org.uk/index.php/contraception/my-contraception-tool/start-my-contraception-tool. It's an online questionnaire that helps you choose the right contraception for you.

Sometimes, I like to compare contraception to shoes. I have size nine feet and I often struggle to find the right pair of shoes that will combine elegance with comfort. Many of us struggle to find the right footwear, but I can confidently say that I haven't seen anyone walking barefoot because they could not find the right pair of shoes!

In the same way, I encourage people to keep searching for their ideal method of contraception. Doing nothing is the worst choice of all because it can have such sad and serious consequences.

Condoms

Condoms are made from different types of rubber or non-rubber material. The **male condom** is worn over the erect penis (like a glove) and it collects the sperm released by the man during sex, preventing its entry into the woman.

Rolled latex condom   Male condom

Squeeze tip of condom so no air
is trapped inside and continue to
hold tip while unrolling condom
to base of penis

The Female Condom

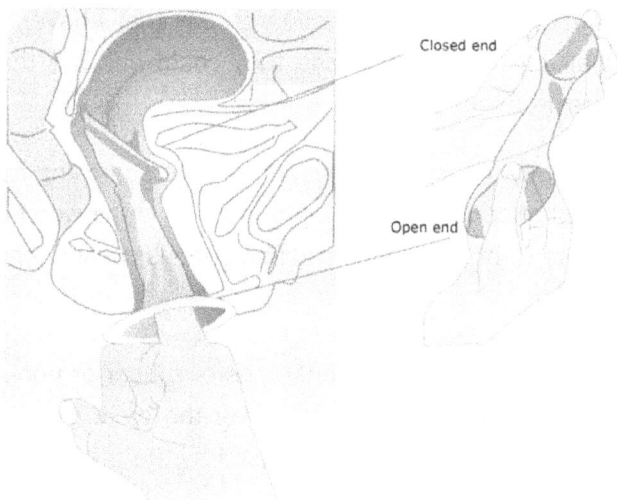

Closed end

Open end

The **female condom** is a bit different. It is inserted into a woman's vagina and sexual intercourse takes place within the condom. Again, any sperm released by the man stays in the bag and cannot go into the womb.

Effectiveness: When used consistently and correctly, male and female condoms are 98% and 95% effective, respectively.

Advantages:

- Condoms are either cheap or free and easily available from sexual health clinics, shops, pharmacists, petrol stations, public toilets, pubs, nightclubs and many other places. A doctor's prescription is not required to buy condoms.

- They have no serious side effects.

- Condoms can help to maintain an erection for longer. This can be useful for men who experience premature ejaculation.

- Male condoms come in a selection of shapes and sizes so most people can find a type that suits them. Using the correct size of condom may decrease the risk of the condom breaking or falling off during sexual intercourse.

- Condoms are only used when having sex so are not in the body at other times.

- Condoms are proven to prevent many sexually transmitted infections such as HIV and should be used in all situations where fidelity is not guaranteed.

- Condoms do not contain hormones.

Disadvantages:

- Can slip off or split during sex.

- Can diminish enjoyment of sex for some.

- Men or their partners may be allergic to the condom's latex.

Helpful Hints

- Do not use oil-based substances like moisturisers or Vaseline as lubricants as they damage condoms. Any additional lubricant increases the risk of slippage.

- Correct sizing can reduce breakage – make sure it is not too tight.

- Breakage rates are the same for standard and "extra strong" condoms so standard ones are all you need.

- There are non-latex options available if you are allergic to latex.

- If you think you have used a condom incorrectly and may be at risk of pregnancy, see your healthcare provider as soon as possible for emergency contraception.

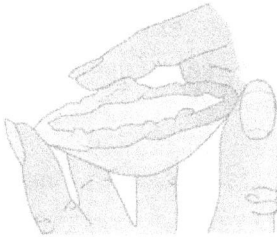

(a)

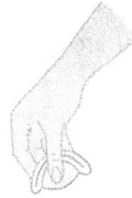

(b)

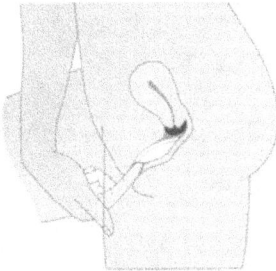

(c)

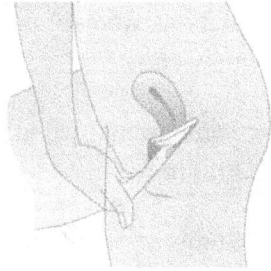

(d)

Cervical caps and diaphragms

These are cap-shaped devices that a woman can fit into her vagina to cover the cervix.

Effectiveness: When used with a spermicide (creams that contain chemicals that kill sperm) they are about 92% effective.

Advantages:

- Same advantages as condoms.

- They can be washed with soap and water and re-used.

Disadvantages:

- A doctor or nurse will have to examine you to ensure that you are given the right sized cap or diaphragm.

- Can be displaced during sexual intercourse if incorrectly inserted or if the wrong size is used. This increases the risk of pregnancy.

- Not all women are comfortable inserting and removing these devices.

- Some women find the devices or even the spermicides irritating.

- Some women find them messy and fiddly, especially when used with spermicides.

- Diaphragms may press on the urethra (the pipe carrying urine to the outside of the body) and this may predispose some women to urine infections.

Caps and diaphragms offer little or no protection against sexually transmitted diseases. They are not recommended for use in situations where there is a high risk of transmission of infection, for example if one's partner has HIV. If these devices are used in these situations, the male partner should also wear male condoms.

Helpful hints

- If you have gained or lost more than 3kg in weight, or have just had a baby, you need to see your doctor or nurse to check that your diaphragm is still the right size for you.

- Women should always check their devices for rips or tears before using them.

- Apply spermicide on the inside of the diaphragm (it doesn't matter if the device is put upside down for most of them but check the instruction leaflet!)

- Spermicides will need to be re-applied if it has been more than three hours since the last application or if you have sex again (you do not need to remove the cap or diaphragm to do this).

- After your last episode of intercourse, the cap or diaphragm needs to stay in place for up to six hours before it is removed. This gives time for any sperm in the vicinity to die off.

Nneka's story

After the birth of their second child, Nneka and her husband decided that their family was complete. They used condoms as their preferred method of contraception and were comfortable with this.

Five years later, Nneka discovered she was pregnant. They were both sure that they had used condoms correctly on every occasion and to this today they still don't know how a pregnancy could have resulted.

She went ahead and had her third child but subsequently came to the sexual health clinic and chose a more effective method of contraception that did not depend on her accurate use.

<hr />

Fertility Fact no. 7

Condoms are up to 98% effective at preventing pregnancy if they are used correctly and consistently.[5]

<hr />

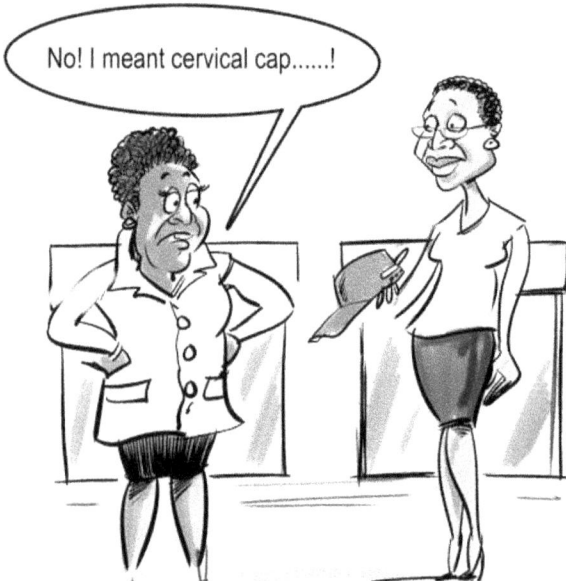

Chapter 6:'Coils?' 'Yes, coils!'

Tobe's story

Tobe had always had heavy periods. Following the birth of her fifth child, she came to see me for contraception. She was particularly interested in a method that would reduce her menstrual bleeding.

After a long discussion, she opted for a hormone containing coil which provided her with very effective contraception for five years and in addition greatly reduced her periods.

Bahati's story

After a very difficult pregnancy complicated by diabetes and hypertension, Bahati was convinced that she didn't want any more pregnancies and asked for a very reliable contraceptive. She didn't want to be sterilised, so she opted for a copper coil which gave her contraceptive cover for 10 years.

It has been known for many centuries that if an object is placed in the womb, it could prevent a pregnancy.

The contraceptive coil is one such object. This chapter deals with this very effective means of contraception.

There are two types of coil available in the UK:

1.   Intrauterine device (IUD, copper coil, "coil").

2.   Intrauterine system (IUS, Mirena® coil).

The main distinction between the two is that the IUD contains copper while the IUS contains a hormone.

Intrauterine device

A copper coil is a small plastic device that has a thread of copper wound round it. It is very small, about the size of a 10 pence coin.

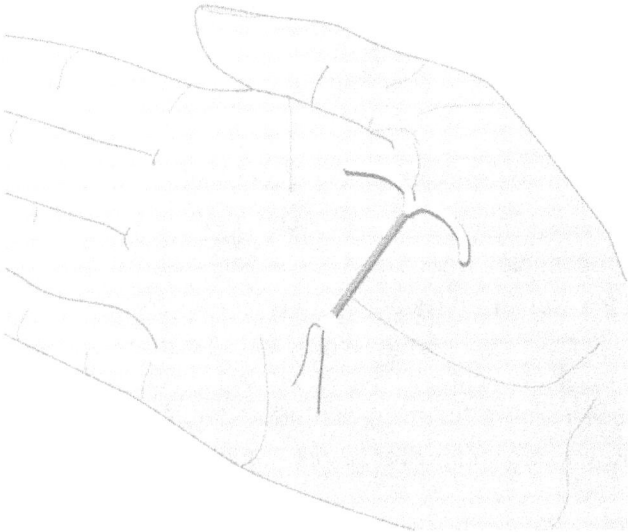

Intrauterine System (IUS, Mirena® coil)

This coil releases a progestogen hormone similar to the hormone progesterone released from women's ovaries.

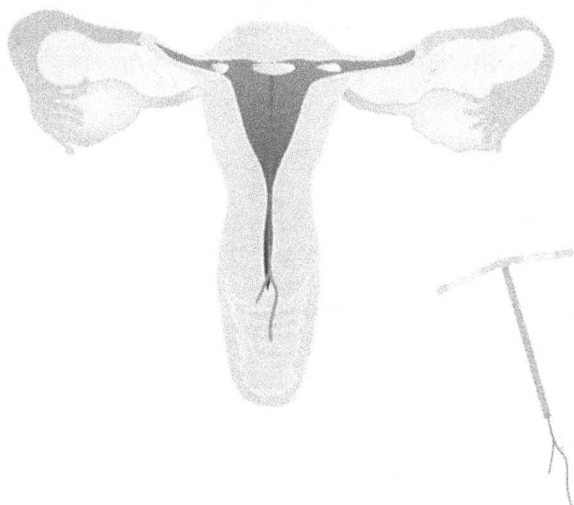

Effectiveness: Both are more than 99% effective at preventing pregnancy.

Coils: the advantages		
IUD	IUS	Both
Works for up to 10 years.	It lasts for five years but can be removed earlier if the woman wishes.	Instantly reversible: you can take it out and get pregnant that month!
It is immediately effective: that is, it starts protecting you against pregnancy once it is put in as long as you are not already pregnant.	It is immediately effective if it is inserted during the first seven days of your period.	It can be inserted at the time of miscarriage or abortion and is immediately effective.
If inserted when you are 40 years and above, you can leave it in until you reach the menopause.	If it is inserted at age 45 or above, you can leave it in until you have reached the menopause.	Can be used if you are breastfeeding.
It does not contain any hormones.	It contains the hormone progesterone which is generally safe to take if you have other health conditions that make it unsafe to take contraception which contain oestrogen.	
It is not affected by other medications you may be taking so can be used by most women regardless of medical history.	It helps prevent anaemia in women with heavy periods.	
	It can make periods lighter and less painful.	

Coils: the disadvantages		
IUD	**IUS**	**Both**
	If it is inserted after day eight of your period, you will need to wait seven days before it becomes effective.	Needs to be fitted by a medical practitioner.
It may initially make periods heavier, longer and more painful, but this usually settles down quickly.	It may cause short-lived hormonal side effects such as breast tenderness, mild headaches and acne.	It might be difficult to fit if you have had any surgeries or treatment to your cervix or if there is a problem with your womb such as huge fibroids.
	It may cause fluid filled swellings on the ovaries. These are not cancers, are not usually harmful, nor require treatment.	Rarely, it may be expelled by the womb.
		Very rarely, the coil may perforate the wall of the womb.
		Does not protect against sexually transmitted infections.

Helpful Hints

- Your contraceptive provider will usually assess your risk of having an infection. This may lead him/her to do some swabs first to avoid introducing bugs into the womb during the process of fitting the coil.

- The coil is gently introduced into the womb through the neck of the womb, like a smear test.

- Although it might be slightly uncomfortable, in my experience most women cope well with it. It is usually over in just 15 minutes.

- You might have a bit of tummy cramp for a short period afterwards as the coil settles into position. Cramping can be eased by taking painkillers like Ibuprofen before the insertion.

Fertility Fact no. 9

The Faculty of Sexual and Reproductive Healthcare clearly states that coils are not abortifacient.[7]
That is, they do not cause abortion.

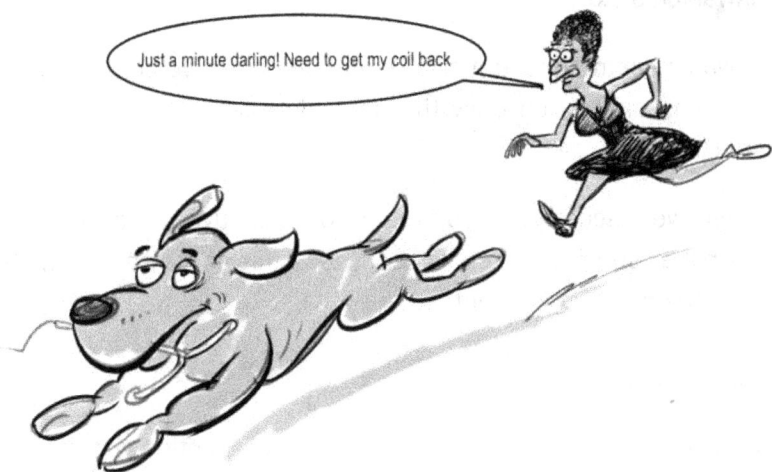

Chapter 7: Pills, patches and rings

Fertility fact no. 10

If 100 women use the pill for a year and none of them
ever forget to take a pill, it's very likely that
none of them will get pregnant.

Akwasiba's story

Akwasiba came to see me to request an effective contraceptive. She was already on daily thyroid tablets to correct her thyroid deficiency.

When we discussed the different contraceptives, she opted for the pill as she felt she could easily take this at the same time as she took her thyroid tablet.

Tamela's story

Tamela had quit smoking with the use of nicotine patches 18 months before she came to see me about contraception. She was pleased to learn of the availability of contraceptive patches which could be used in a similar way to nicotine patches.

She found these easy and convenient to use until she was ready to start a family four years later.

Ibifaa's story

Ibifaa has been using contraceptive rings for many years. She comes regularly to collect her rings and has found them convenient and easy to use. She is particularly pleased that she doesn't need a doctor or nurse to help her fit the ring.

Combined pills, patches and rings all contain two hormones – an oestrogen and a progestogen.

Combined pills ('the pill')

These are very popular and an effective means of contraception. Most pills are taken daily for three weeks and then there is a week's break during which you have a bleed. It is important to re-start your pill immediately after the week-long break even if you are still bleeding, otherwise you will lose your contraceptive cover.

Contraceptive Pill

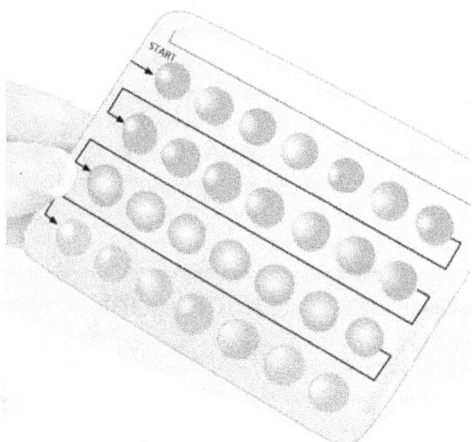

Contraceptive Patch

This is applied weekly for three weeks and then a patch-free week follows when no patch is worn and a period comes. It is important to remember to put on a new patch after the seven day patch-free period whether you are bleeding or not, otherwise you will lose your contraceptive cover.

The contraceptive patch can be placed anywhere except the breasts.

Contraceptive Patch

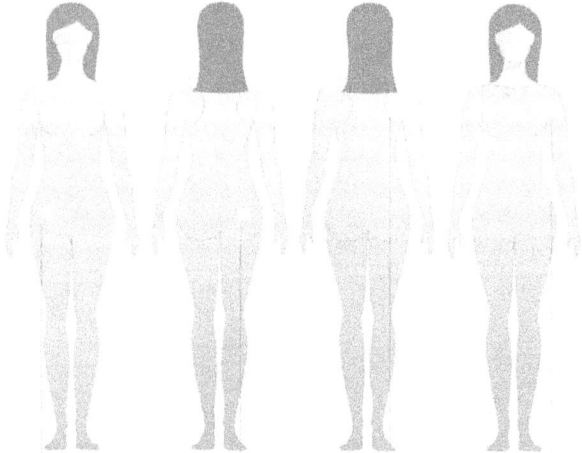

Helpful Hint

Most women apply the patch to their buttocks, abdomen, upper outer arm or back.

Contraceptive ring

A ring the size of a small pony tail band is inserted into the vagina, stays for three weeks and then is removed. A seven-day ring-free period then follows after which another ring is inserted.

Again, as with the patch and the pill, you must remember to put in another ring after the ring-free period whether you are bleeding or not, otherwise you will lose your contraceptive cover. The ring is usually self-inserted, poses no danger to your partner and does not have to be positioned in any particular way in the vagina.

Contraceptive Ring

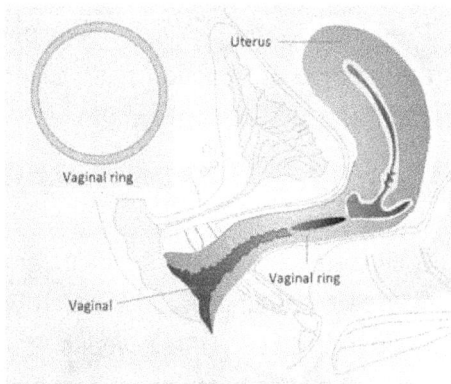

Effectiveness: Used consistently and correctly, they are all more than 99% effective.

Advantages:

- They make periods lighter and less painful.

- They help regularise an erratic period.

- They do not interfere with sex as you are not required to take them out at the time of intercourse.

- They reduce the risk of some types of cancers such as cancer of the womb, ovary and colon.

- Can reduce the development of non-cancerous breast lumps.

- They thicken the cervical mucus and this may help reduce the chance of infection getting into the womb. They may improve premenstrual symptoms.

Disadvantages:

- You need to be really good at remembering to take your pills daily, putting on your patch weekly or inserting your vaginal ring every three weeks. If you are forgetful, these may not be the best options for you.

- Research suggests that there is a slightly greater risk of developing breast and cervical cancer compared with those who don't take hormones.

- They are not suitable for smokers over the age of 35 or for very overweight women.

- They may not be suitable for you if you have certain health problems.

- They can cause hormonal side effects like nausea, moodiness, breast tenderness or headaches. Many other women taking these preparations do not experience any of these side effects or find that they are quite mild. Side effects often diminish as you take the pill. Consult your doctor as there are usually other options you could try if you are finding the side effects unbearable.

- There is a very small risk of developing a blood clot, or having a heart attack or stroke while using them.

- They can also cause an increase in blood pressure, so make sure to have a blood pressure check at three months and subsequently as advised by your doctor.

The progesterone only pill (POP, mini-pill)

The POP is a contraceptive pill which releases a progestogen hormone.

Helpful Hint

You may wish to omit the pill/patch/ring-free week and just keep taking the pill/patch/ring if you wish to avoid a bleed.

Nneoma's story

Nneoma, a 37-year-old accountant, wanted to take 'the pill'. An obese lady with a body mass index (BMI) of 41, she had recently been found to have high blood pressure. Due to her weight and blood pressure, it was medically unsafe to give her the combined pill.

We discussed other contraceptives but she felt a pill was the most convenient method for her. I therefore started her on the 'mini-pill' which is safe as it does not contain any oestrogen contraindicated in her situation.

Effectiveness: It is more than 99% effective when used consistently and correctly.

| Progesterone only pills 'mini-pill' : for and against ||
Advantages	Disadvantages
Can be used in women who are unable to take the oestrogen for medical reasons.	Must be taken every day.
Can be used while breast feeding.	Hormonal side effects such as nausea, breast tenderness and headaches.
It can be used by obese ladies and by smokers.	Up to 40% of women will experience erratic bleeding.
May ease premenstrual symptoms and painful periods (some women find their periods stop while taking the POP).	Research suggests that all hormonal contraception may result in a slight increase in breast cancer.
Doesn't cause weight changes, headache or depression.	No protection against sexually transmitted infections.

Fertility Fact no. 11
In Nigeria, the number of maternal deaths per 100,000 live births is 840. This compares to 24 in the US and 12 in the UK.[8]

Chapter 8: There are injections and implants as well!

> **Fertility Fact no. 12**
> Of women aged between 15-49, only 2% of Nigerian women use the contraceptive injection compared to 28% in South Africa.[9]

Contraceptive Injection

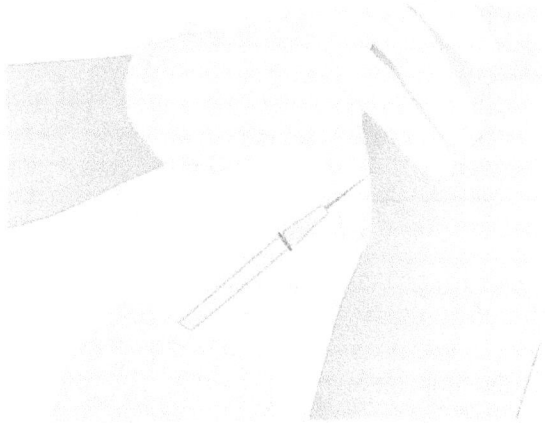

The contraceptive injection releases a progestogen hormone.

Effectiveness: more than 99% effective at preventing pregnancy.

Advantages:

- Does not interfere with sex.

- May help premenstrual symptoms, excess menstrual blood loss and mid-cycle (ovulation) and period pain (dysmenorrhoea).

- Treats endometriosis, which gets worse with periods.

- Can reduce fits if epileptic and decrease sickling or painful crises in women with sickle cell disease.

- It can be used when breastfeeding.

- Not affected by other medications.

- It is long acting; protects against pregnancy for three months following each injection.

Handy hint

It is injected into your buttock or arm.

Disadvantages :

- Can cause weight gain. This risk can be reduced by increasing physical activity and eating smaller food portions.

- It cannot be removed once it is injected. Therefore if you are having any side effects, you will have to wait for the effect of the hormone to wear off.

- It can delay the return of periods and fertility for up to one year after stopping.

- It may lead to a slight thinning of the bones which reverses if you stop using it. To help counteract this, women on the injection are advised to stay physically active, to eat/drink calcium containing foods and to avoid smoking. However, it may not be suitable if you have additional risks of bone thinning.

- It can only be given as an injection.

- In some women, it can cause periods to be unpredictable (irregular, heavier or lighter) especially in the first few months of use. After a year, up to 70% of women will have no bleeding which may be a good or bad thing depending on your point of view. If no periods result, money is saved on sanitary protection, anaemia is prevented and it's easier to manage personal hygiene.

- As seen in other hormonal contraceptives, hormonal side effects may occur.

- Does not protect against sexually transmitted infections.

- Research suggests that all hormonal contraception may result in a slight increase in breast cancer.

Adowa's story

Adowa, an 18 year-old-lady with sickle cell disease, came with her mum to request contraception. She did not think she would remember to take tablets daily. She also preferred a contraceptive that would take her periods away as they were painful, heavy and accompanied by mood swings.

I discussed several methods with her. She didn't mind needles and so opted for injectables. I explained that seven in 10 people on injectables do not have periods. She was happy to hear this as she often got anaemic due to her sickle cell condition and heavy periods.

She received her first injection after a check to ensure that she was not pregnant. I invited her to return to the nurse 12 weeks later to have her next injection, or earlier if she had any problems she wished to discuss.

Fertility Fact no. 13

Contraceptive injections are so effective that only four women in a 1000 will get pregnant over two years of use.

Chapter 9: The contraceptive implant

This is called Nexplanon in the UK. It is a small rod which can be inserted into the inner arm under local anaesthesia. Like the injection, it releases a progestogen hormone.

Nexplanon

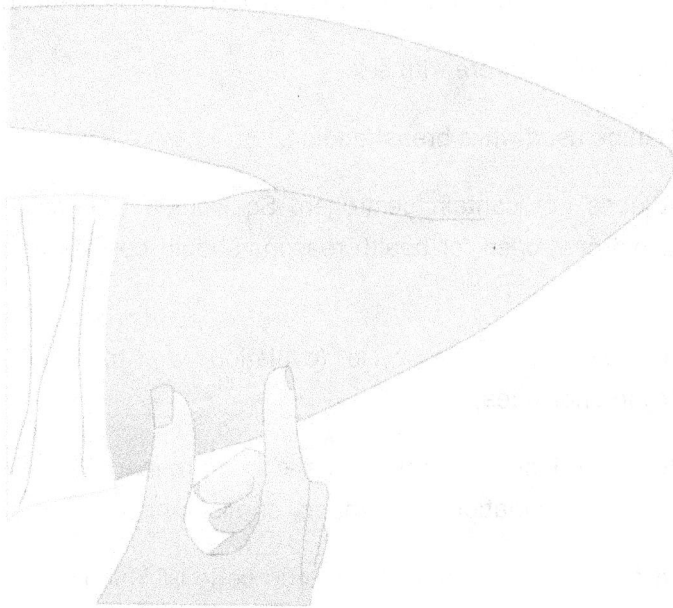

Effectiveness: It is more than 99% effective at preventing pregnancy.

> **Fertility Fact no. 14**
> Less than one woman in every 1000 will get pregnant over three years using the implant.

Advantages:

- It is long acting – protects against pregnancy for three years.

- It can be removed any time and fertility returns immediately.

- It doesn't interfere with sex.

- Can be used while breastfeeding.

- It does not contain oestrogen. So women who have to avoid oestrogen for health reasons should be safe to use it.

- It may improve mid-cycle (ovulation) and period pain (dysmenorrhoea).

- It can be inserted three weeks after a pregnancy or at the time of termination of pregnancy or miscarriage.

- In one in five women, it can stop periods. This is a great advantage to women who normally bleed heavily or suffer from painful periods.

Disadvantages:

- Periods become unpredictable (infrequent, frequent or prolonged) in about half of women. With perseverance, many find that their periods eventually regularise or go away completely so it's worth giving the implant six months to see if things settle down.

- There can be a small amount of bruising, scarring or infection at the site of insertion of the implant.

- It needs to be fitted and removed by a trained professional.

- As seen in other hormonal contraceptives, temporary side effects such as skin changes and breast tenderness may occur.

- All hormonal contraception appears to confer a small increase in risk of breast cancer.

- Some drugs interfere with the implant.

- Does not protect against STIs.

Ijeoma's story

Ijeoma, a 28-year-old nurse, wanted a contraceptive method which would be effective, easy to use and would not require any effort on her part. Due to her shift pattern of work, she felt she would struggle to use any method daily.

We discussed all the methods and she opted for the contraceptive implant. This was easily inserted and would give her contraceptive cover for three years which she was delighted to hear.

Fertility Fact no.15

There are 970 maternal deaths per 100,000 live births in Sierra Leone, Africa compared with five maternal deaths per 100,000 live births in Sweden.[10]

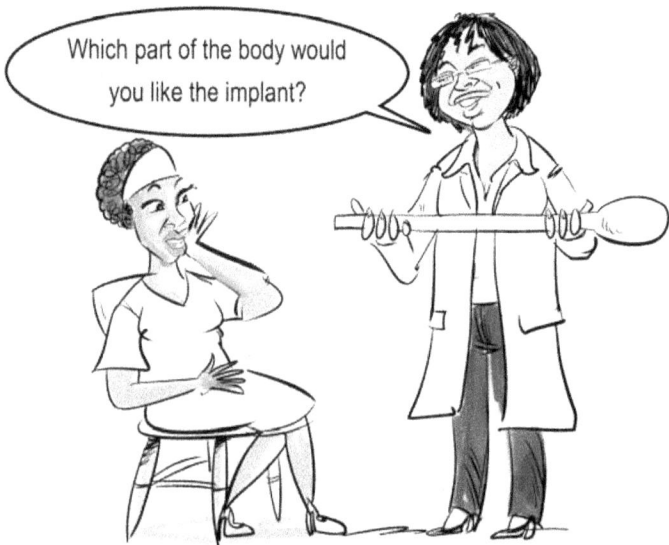

Chapter 10: Sterilisation

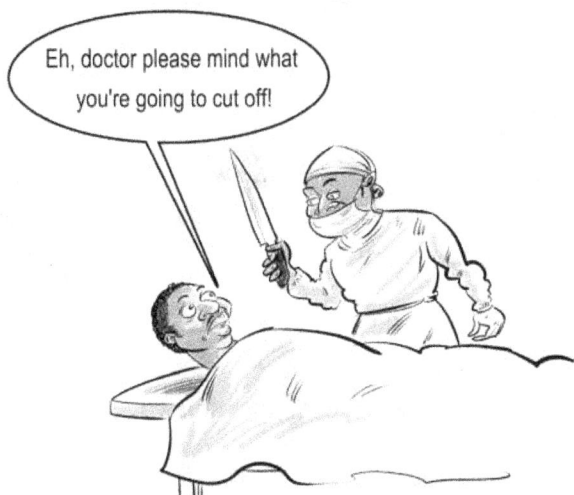

Eh, doctor please mind what you're going to cut off!

Fertility Fact no. 16

Male sterilisation rates in Sierra Leone is 0% compared to 22% in Canada and 19% in New Zealand.[11]

Chimanda's story

Chimanda and her husband Obinna had completed their family and came to request a permanent method of contraception. She had tried a number of different contraceptives but now wanted something that would ensure that she never needed to worry about pregnancy again.

We discussed both male and female sterilisations. They went home to think about what they wanted. At the next appointment, Obinna informed me he wanted to be sterilised. This was arranged and they are both very pleased with their choice.

Sterilisation is a procedure which can be carried out on a male or female with the sole purpose of achieving **PERMANENT** contraception.

Female sterilisation

Sterilisation can be done in several ways but the underlying principle is that the tubes that carry the eggs are tied, clipped or blocked in order to prevent the transfer of eggs down the tube or sperm up the tube.

If the sperm and egg cannot meet, a pregnancy cannot result. It can be done under general or local anaesthesia.

Effectiveness: It is more than 99% effective in preventing pregnancy.

Laparoscopic Female Sterilization

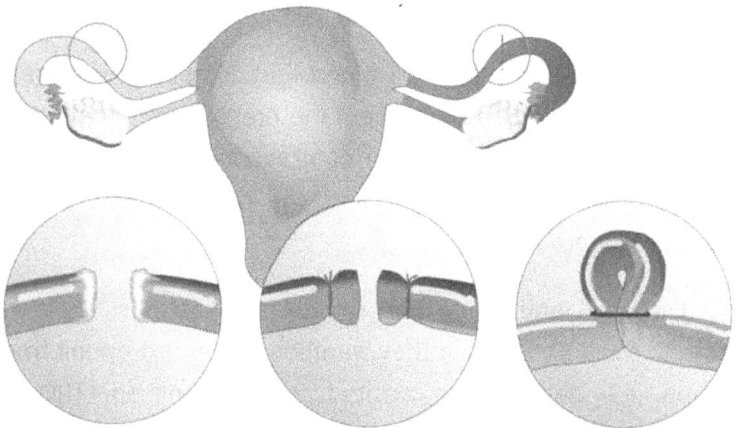

Cauterized   Tied and cut   Banded

Helpful hints

Female sterilisation can be an 'open surgery' in which a cut is made into the abdomen and under direct vision, the two tubes are tied/clipped or cut. This can be done at the time of caesarean section. More often, though, sterilisation is done as 'keyhole surgery' where small cuts are made on the tummy and special equipment introduced to make a block in the tubes. This is called laparoscopic sterilisation and is quicker to recover from than the open operation.

More recently, a simpler procedure is now being done where small 'micro-inserts' (like springs) are passed into the tubes from the vagina. This avoids the need for any cuts on the tummy or general anaesthesia. It is called Hysteroscopic Sterilisation.

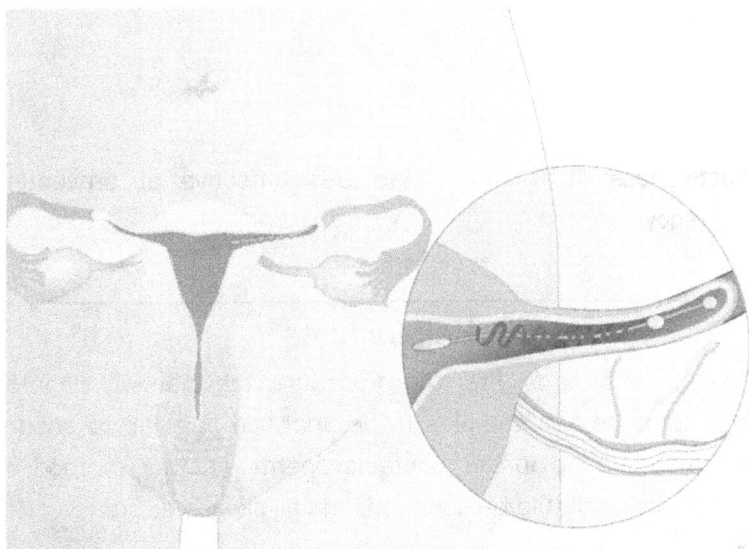

Male sterilisation (vasectomy)

Vasectomy involves a simple procedure whereby the tubes that carry sperm are cut under local or general anaesthesia. This means that when a man comes, the fluid no longer contains sperm and so cannot fertilise a woman's eggs.

Male Vasectomy

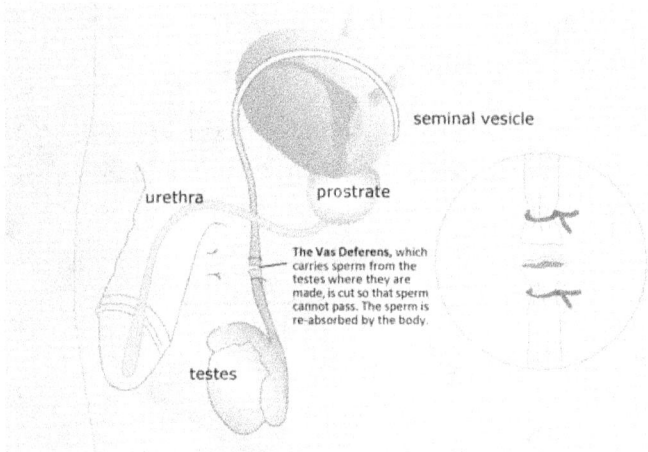

seminal vesicle

urethra

prostrate

The Vas Deferens, which carries sperm from the testes where they are made, is cut so that sperm cannot pass. The sperm is re-absorbed by the body.

testes

Effectiveness: It is more than 99% effective at preventing pregnancy.

Helpful hints

A couple of months after the procedure, the man will need to send some semen samples to be analysed in a lab to ensure that the fluid no longer contains sperm. Another method of contraception should be used until the all clear is given.

Advantages:

- You won't need to use contraception again.

Disadvantages:

- Both procedures are meant to be permanent and attempts to reverse them are usually unsuccessful. Therefore there may be regrets if the decision to go for sterilisation is not carefully thought through. About 5% of people regret their decision to be sterilised.

- There are rare cases where the tubes rejoin. This makes you (or your partner) fertile again.

- It does not protect against STIs.

Possible risks you need to know

Male sterilisation

- The procedure can result in bleeding, infection or swelling which settle in time.

- Very occasionally, a vasectomy causes ongoing pain in the testicles.

<u>Female Sterilisation</u>

- If the procedure is keyhole, damage to blood vessels or other organs may result.

- There is a small increased risk of ectopic pregnancy (pregnancy outside the womb, usually in the tubes).

Fertility Fact no. 17

Female sterilisation rate in Nigeria is only 0.2% compared to 22% in USA and 13% in UK.[12]

Chapter 11: Emergency and traditional methods of contraception

Emergency contraception (EC)

This is very useful in situations where contraception has not been used or has failed. This would include such situations as a burst condom. In the UK, EC can be obtained free from pharmacies, sexual health clinics, and from your general practitioner.

Emergency contraception takes the form of either tablets or the copper IUD (coil). While the coil is the most effective, if the tablet form is chosen it should be taken as soon as possible.

Traditional methods of contraception

Traditional methods are still practiced by many and include withdrawal, checking the consistency of cervical mucus, taking your temperature daily and so on. These are discussed fully in other literature.[13] The efficacy of these methods depends on your age, how often you are having sex, and how consistently you follow the method's instructions.

Helpful Hint

As traditional methods have a much higher failure rate than modern contraceptives, they should only be used if you do not mind getting pregnant.

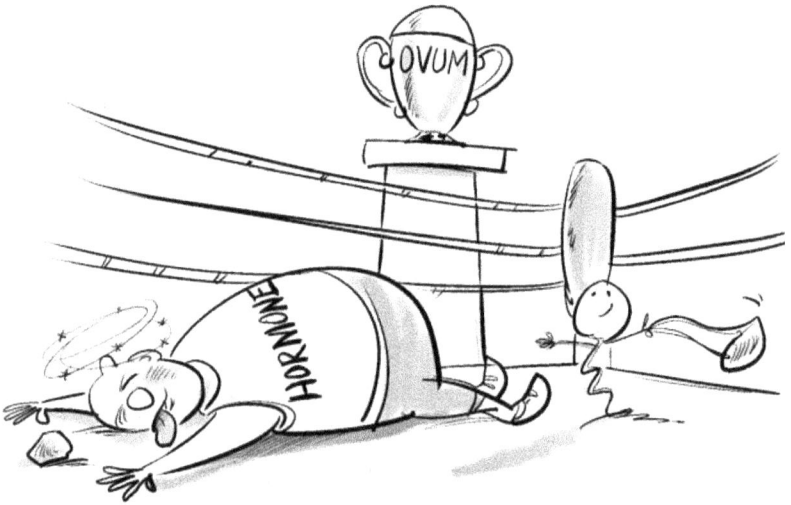

Chapter 12: What to expect from your contraception provider in the UK

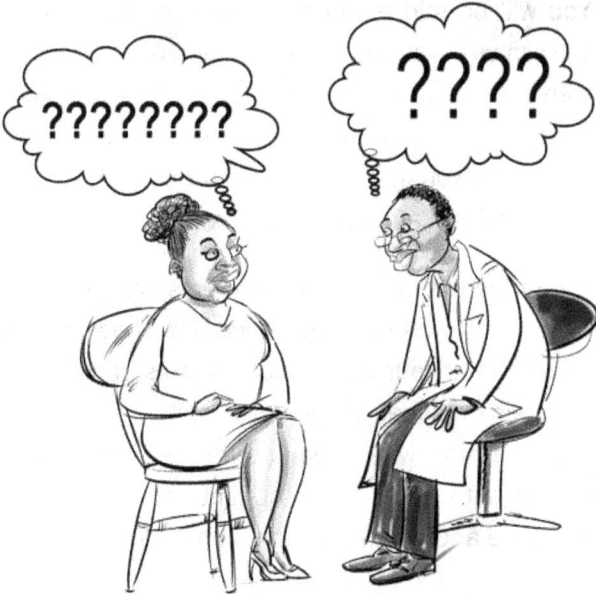

Many foreign ladies are embarrassed and apprehensive about attending clinics for contraception. They worry about being judged or criticised by medical staff. Language or communication difficulties are also reasons for low uptake of services by immigrant ladies.

The information below will hopefully allay some of these concerns and encourage greater uptake of sexual health services by migrants.

• **You can request the use of 'language line'** when you attend either a specialist contraceptive service or your GP if you think that communicating in English will be a problem. This service ensures that an interpreter who speaks your language can be available by phone.

- **You will be told about all the contraception methods** that you can use, how they work and any risks or benefits associated with them. You will be allowed to make the choice that is suitable for you. It may not be easy for you to decide what is best for you in just one appointment, so you can ask for another if you are still undecided.

- **Do not be put off when side effects are discussed.** You are more likely to tolerate side effects if you have been forewarned about them. Your views and concerns about contraception, whether personal, religious or cultural, will be taken into consideration when you attend the clinic. Your nurse or doctor will explore your thoughts and circumstances in a sensitive and non-judgemental manner.

- **Contraception will not be forced on you** even if it would benefit your health.

- **You might want to encourage your partner to come with you.** Women are more likely to continue to use contraception if their partners are involved in the decision to use it.

- **The clinic will want to see you again if you are having any problems.** All clinics operate an open door policy that encourages a woman to come back if her contraception does not suit her.

- **Unnecessary delays can lead to unplanned pregnancy,** so once you have decided on a contraceptive, your clinic will make every effort to provide this or refer you to where you can get the contraception.

- **Any information you share with your doctor or nurse will be kept confidential** unless he or she thinks that disclosing this information will be in your best interest or in the public interest. In that case, your consent will be sought.

- **All contraception, including sterilisation, is provided FREE OF CHARGE by the NHS.**

Acknowledgements

This book would not have been possible without the support and input of friends, family and colleagues.

Heartfelt thanks to Dr Susie Logan, Consultant Gynaecologist and sexual health expert, for her encouragement and suggestions. Thank you for taking the time to read through to ensure that the information used in the book is medically sound.

My husband, Chigbo Ifezulike, thank you for believing in me and for your endless patience and support.

My lovely children for their support and love.

My parents, Dr Michael and Pauline Ogbalu, whose constant enquiry about the book spurred me on when I grew a bit weary.

Jane Mallin for her painstaking proof reading and editing of the book. Jane, your advice and constant feedback were invaluable.

Chris Day and the Filament team for producing an excellent work.

To my patients whose stories have formed the bedrock of this book, I say 'thank you'.

My love and gratitude to my beloved siblings (the Ogbalu Octet) who always inspire me to be the best that I can be.

My BFF Dr Blessing Okpo, you never doubted I could do it. Thanks.

Dr John Duncan, a man of excellence who sowed the invaluable seeds of professionalism in me during my training as a family physician under him, thanks.

Thanks to Pastor Iyiola Ogedengbe, Dr Joyce Otakoro, Dr Ronnie Okafor and the RCCG Higher Ground parish at Westhill, Aberdeenshire.

Thanks to Pastor Mark Igiehon, Ngozi Vincent-Eloagu, Tolu Olowoleru and other dear friends at the children's church RCCG, Jesus House, Aberdeen.

To friends and family who helped in one way or another, many thanks.

References

Chapter 1:

1. Abortion statistics 2012, England and Wales Department of Health.
2. *The Telegraph*, 'Abortion costs £30m higher than previously thought', 22 Nov 2011.

Chapter 4:

3. Jones, RK, 'Beyond Birth Control: The Overlooked Benefits Of Oral Contraceptive Pills'. New York: Guttmacher Institute, 2011
4. World Population data sheet 2010. (Accessed 16/09/2013).

Chapter 5:

5. FSRH Male and female condoms, Clinical effectiveness unit. January 2007 http://www.fsrh.org/pdfs/archive/CEUguidanceMaleFemaleCondomsJan07.pdf. (Accessed 16/09/ 2013).

Chapter 6:

6. World population data sheet 2012. (Accessed 16/09/2013).
7. FSRH Intrauterine Contraception, Clinical Effectiveness Unit. November2007 http://www.fsrh.org/pdfs/CEUGuidanceIntrauterineContraceptionNov07.pdf. (Accessed 16/09/2013).

Chapter 7:

8.   World population data sheet 2012. (Accessed 16/09/2013).

Chapter 8:

9.   World population data sheet 2012. (Accessed 16/09/ 2013).

Chapter 9:

10.   World population data sheet 2012. (Accessed 16/09/ 2013).

Chapter 10:

11.   World population data sheet 2012. (Accessed 16/09/2013).

12.   World population data sheet 2012. (Accessed 16/09/ 2013).

Chapter 11:

13.   http://www.fpa.org.uk/product/natural-family-planning-contraceptive-methods-booklets.

Useful contacts

NHS Direct: www.nhsdirect.nhs.uk.
Telephone 0845 4647.

NHS 24: 0845 4242424.

Brook: www.brook.org.uk

Family Planning Association: www.fpa.org.uk

Rape and Sexual Abuse Support Centre: www.rapecrisis.org.uk
Freephone helpline 0808 802 9999.

Rape Crisis Scotland Helpline 0808 801 0302.

Your local GP's surgery

Your local pharmacy

Appendix 1

Chart comparing effectiveness of all contraceptives.

Effectiveness of Contraceptive Methods

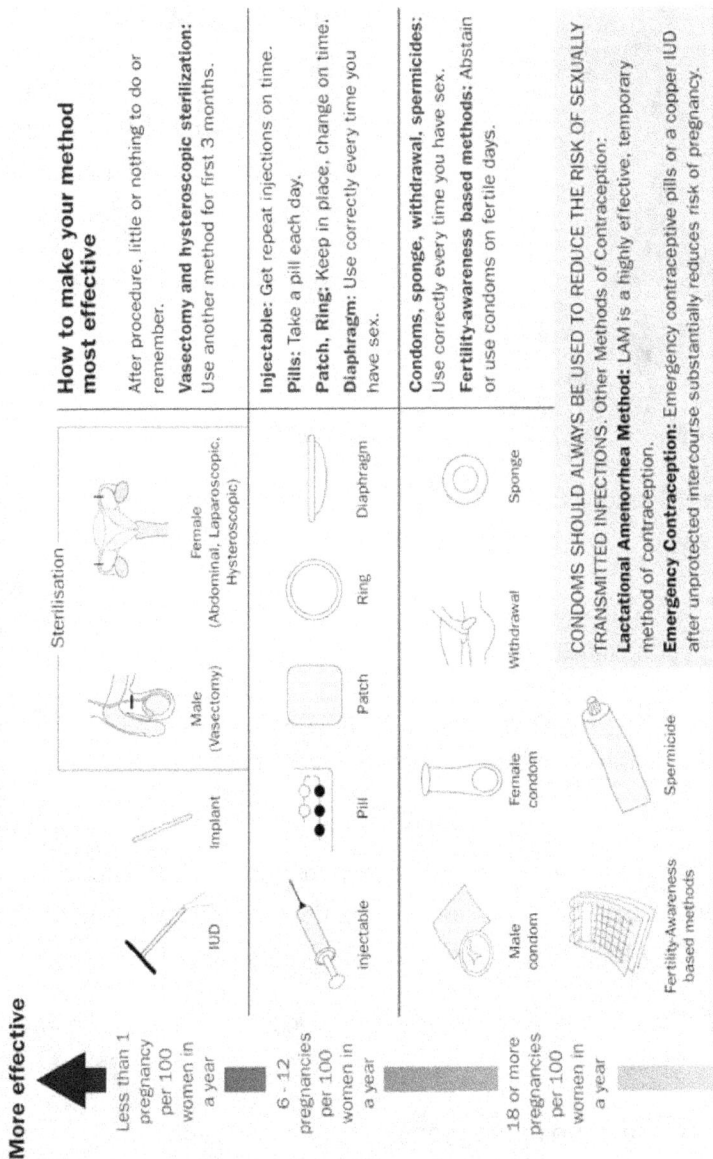

More effective

	How to make your method most effective
Sterilisation — Male (Vasectomy), Female (Abdominal, Laparoscopic, Hysteroscopic)	After procedure, little or nothing to do or remember. **Vasectomy and hysteroscopic sterilization:** Use another method for first 3 months.

Less than 1 pregnancy per 100 women in a year

IUD, Implant

6 - 12 pregnancies per 100 women in a year

injectable, Pill, Patch, Ring, Diaphragm

- **Injectable:** Get repeat injections on time.
- **Pills:** Take a pill each day.
- **Patch, Ring:** Keep in place, change on time.
- **Diaphragm:** Use correctly every time you have sex.

18 or more pregnancies per 100 women in a year

Male condom, Female condom, Withdrawal, Sponge, Fertility-Awareness based methods, Spermicide

- **Condoms, sponge, withdrawal, spermicides:** Use correctly every time you have sex.
- **Fertility-awareness based methods:** Abstain or use condoms on fertile days.

CONDOMS SHOULD ALWAYS BE USED TO REDUCE THE RISK OF SEXUALLY TRANSMITTED INFECTIONS. Other Methods of Contraception: **Lactational Amenorrhea Method:** LAM is a highly effective, temporary method of contraception. **Emergency Contraception:** Emergency contraceptive pills or a copper IUD after unprotected intercourse substantially reduces risk of pregnancy.

Adapted from WHO's Family Planning: A Global Handbook for Providers (2001) and Trussell et al (2011).

Less effective

Adaeze Ifezulike

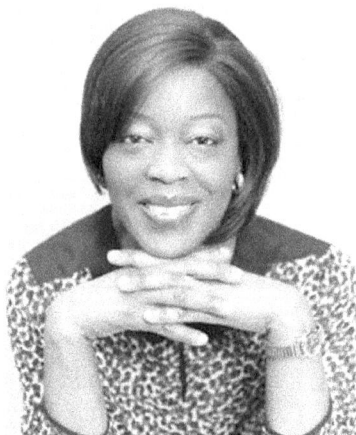

Family Physician / GP / Speaker / Author / Blogger at sexualwellbeing network.org

Expert on how to make better sexual health choices and enjoy a happier and more fulfilled life.

Founder: Sexual Wellbeing Network.

Dubbed "Sexual Wellbeing Champion"

Adaeze Ifezulike is a Family Physician/GP whose empathy and professionalism is an instant hit with audiences of all sizes.

Her speeches are clear, easily understood and delivered to achieve maximum impact.

Humorous, power packed and energetic, Adaeze leaves her audience feeling inspired and ready to take the necessary steps to improve their lives.

She has more than 15 years' experience and knowledge as a medical doctor and infuses her experiences into key life strategies and powerful presentations.

She helps ladies pinpoint areas of focus necessary to create a fulfilling life.

Her seminars are relevant and full of rich content.

Drawing from her own experiences and encounters with patients, she shares effective solutions for maximising life and actionable takeaways that clients can begin to put to use immediately.

Adaeze's ideal audience is women who feel they can be more than they are at present, women with big dreams but who feel limited by self-imposed or society imposed obstacles.

She also loves to share strategies with youths on how they can cultivate their teenage and early adult lives to ensure that they position themselves for greatness.

When you listen to Adaeze, you will see the 'impossible' become possible.

The following is a sample of Speaking Topics that Dr Adaeze Ifezulike is constantly asked to present to groups and organisations. If you are wondering about a topic which isn't listed here, please contact talksexualwellbeing@yahoo.com

Speaking Topics

Domestic Abuse:'No more one-in-four!'

- Get equipped to help a friend who is being abused.

- Gain skills on managing domestic abuse.

Are you the 'one in four' woman? One in four women are victims of domestic abuse.

Are you desperate not to be one of the three women who die daily worldwide from domestic abuse?

Maybe your friend is a victim of domestic abuse. How can you help her?

Join Adaeze Ifezulike as she tackles this cancer with expertise and empathy.

My Dream Man:

- Must-do strategies to position yourself to attract Mr Right.

- The big mistakes that single ladies make.

- What to do while 'waiting' for Mr Right.

Have you been single and ready for so long that you're almost ready to give up on your 'Dream Man'? Do you dream of marital bliss and look forward to your own happily ever after with the man of your dreams?

Are you sick of hearing how terrible marriage is and determined to create your own version of beauty in marriage?

Join Adaeze Ifezulike - Sexual Wellbeing expert - and learn how to make your dreams a reality!

Sexual Intimacy:

- Still wondering what the big deal is about sex?

- Struggling to find sexual fulfilment with your partner?

Adaeze Ifezulike will explore the ways we shoot ourselves in the foot when it comes to sex and strategies for optimising sexual intimacy.

Contraception:

- Is your family complete and you want to stop child-bearing?

- Maybe you are not ready for a family yet and just want some insight on what contraception to use?

- Do you get confused about the different contraceptions and how they work?

- Do you have reservations about their side effects?

Invite Dr Adaeze for a heart-to-heart in-depth analysis on the use of contraception. Learn how to minimise the chance of your chosen contraception failing and discover the truth about side effects like cancer which have been attributed to contraception.

Pornography.

What's so terrible about pornography? It's just looking at pictures. No one gets hurt by me looking at pictures... do they?

Dr Adaeze skilfully handles this explosive issue and

- Equips people with the knowledge they need to deal with pornography.

- Shows a step by step method on how to stop using it.

Making my teenage years count.

Teenage years are the season for sowing and must be deliberately harnessed if one hopes for a great future.

Dr Adaeze's messages to young people will light a fire in their hearts and help them to achieve their greatest potential.

- Learn the pitfalls to success in life.

- Understand how to position yourself for greatness.

The above is just a selection of frequently requested talks (Hot Topics). Other topics can be handled – please email info@sexualwellbeingnetwork.com to enquire about your topic.